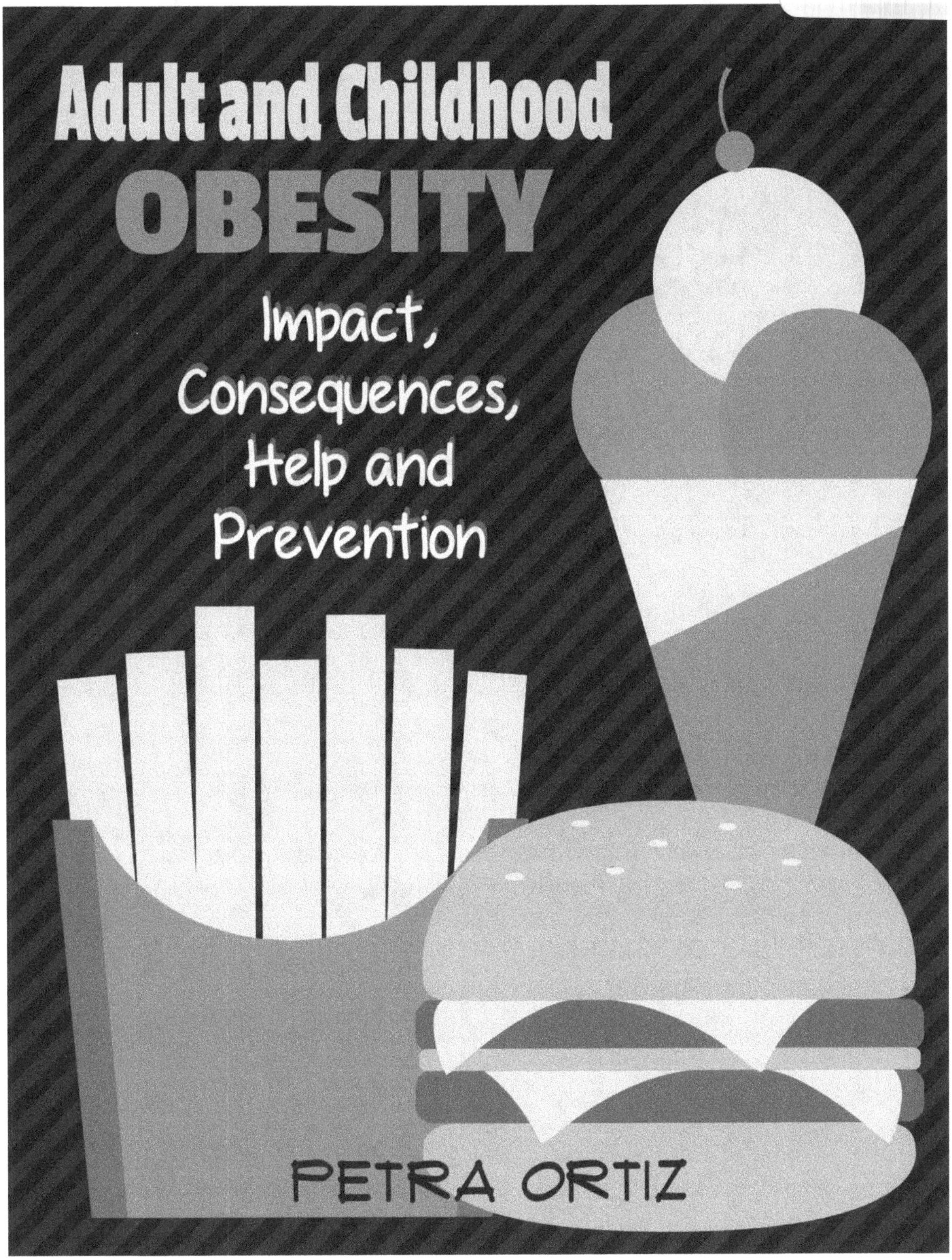

Adult and Childhood
OBESITY

Impact, Consequences, Help and Prevention

PETRA ORTIZ

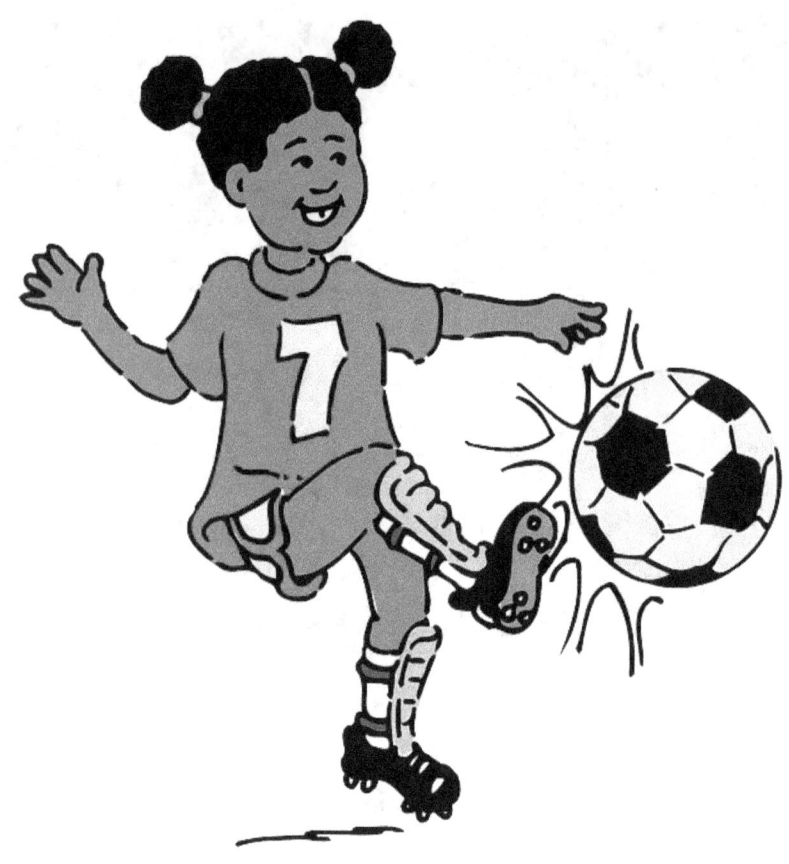

ISBN-13: 978-1502726056
ISBN-10: 150272605X

TABLE OF CONTENTS

What Is Obesity?

Obesity is a medical condition where persons have too much body fat that is difficult to control through dieting and can be contributed to by both genetic and environmental factors. Obesity is identified when one has a Body Mass Index (BMI) of 30 or greater. The American Medical Association classified it as a disease in 2013.

How Obesity Is Measured In Adults

For the most part, clinicians use the Body Mass Index (BMI) measurement to ascertain weight problems and obesity (see image below).
The Body Mass Index (BMI)
According to the CDC, the Body Mass Index (BMI) is a number that is calculated using a person's weight and height.
It provides a reliable indicator of body fat for most people and is used as a screening tool to categorize weight scales that may lead to health problems.
The BMI measurement applies to both men and women.

How Obesity Is Measured In Children

The Center for Disease Control offers growth charts for medical professionals that are used to determine BMI corresponding to age and sex percentiles in kids age 2 to 19.
In kids, overweight is defined as a BMI at or above the 85th percentile, but, below, the 95th percentile for kids of the same age and sex.
Obesity is defined as a BMI at or above the 95th percentile.

BMI Chart For Adults

A BMI of 30 or greater is obese.
A BMI of 40 or greater is considered extreme obesity, also referred to as morbid obesity.

There are charts and also many online calculators to measure BMI. Finding out if you fall into the overweight, obese or extremely obese classification is the beginning step in addressing your weight problems. Any unhealthy range is important to address, and begin the road to good health by speaking with your doctor.

Locate a BMI calculator at
www.pinterest.com/petralovesbats/childhood-obesity

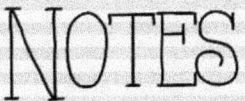

NOTES

The Statistics

Adult Numbers

Obesity is a worldwide problem, and rates of obesity have doubled since 2008 from 15% to 30%.
In the United States, obesity has been deemed an epidemic by the president, due to the record numbers of obesity in both children and adults.
In fact, 68.5% of the US population is either overweight or obese with more than 2/3 of adults being overweight or obese in 2014.
And, 6.4% of the US population are extremely obese with a BMI of 40 or greater.
Worldwide, the number of overweight and obese individuals rose more than 145% from 857 million in 1980 to 2.1 billion in 2013 (Global Burden of Disease Study 2013, published in The Lancet).

Child Numbers

Obesity in children has skyrocketed over the last few years. According to the Centers For Disease Control, from 1980 to 2012 the number of obese kids, ages 6 to 11, has increased from 7% to 18%.

And amongst teens age 12 to 19, from 5% to 21%.

31.8% of adolescents and children are either overweight or obese, and, of those, 16.9% of kids are obese.

1/3 of school age children are obese.

And, ¼ of 2 to 5 year old kids are obese or overweight.

Obesity is a major problem in low income households, where 30.4% of preschoolers are overweight or obese.

By State

Mississippi has the **highest** rates of obesity at 35.4%.
States with the **lowest** rates of obesity are:
- ❖ Montana at 19.6%
- ❖ Colorado at 20.4%
- ❖ Nevada at 21.1%

By Country

More than half of the world's obese individuals live in these ten countries.

1. United States (more than 13%)
2. China
3. India
4. Russia
5. Brazil
6. Mexico
7. Egypt
8. Germany
9. Pakistan
10. Indonesia

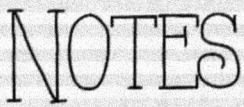

NOTES

Health Consequences Of Obesity

Adults

Obesity is a very serious medical condition that can lead to a variety of health conditions and early death.

Research published in the American Journal of Public Health reports that 18% of all deaths in the United States are attributed to obesity related conditions, which is three times the numbers previously reported by various government sources.

It is also the cause of billions of dollars in health care costs, where those conditions account for more than ¼ of all health care costs in the United States.

When an individual is obese, they are at risk for several different serious health problems. Some of which can be lethal.

The diabetes rates are astounding since 44% of 100% preventable diabetes (Type 2 Diabetes) conditions are attributed to obesity.

99% of all diabetes cases are Type 2 Diabetes, which are preventable and caused by poor diet and obesity, as opposed, to the type people are born with.

23% of all heart disease in the United States is attributed to obesity.

Also, 7% to 41% of specific cancers are obesity related, including, breast (post-menopausal), endometrial and colon cancers.

Life expectancy is shortened by 6 years for the obese and by 10 years for the morbidly obese.

Heart Disease

Obese people have a lot more chance of becoming a victim of abnormal heart rhythm, congestive heart failure, heart attack, and sudden cardiac death.

Obese adolescents too are at greater risk of falling prey to heart attack *before they reach the age 35.*

Reducing weight by 10 to 15 pounds usually decreases the risk of heart disease.

High Blood Pressure

High blood pressure, or hypertension, accounts for the most number of deaths of Americans above the age of 25.

Even though the mechanism behind the increase of blood pressure in obese people is presently unknown, we have enough data to assert that blood pressure increases with an increase in bodyweight; researchers have shown that obese people display arterial resistance and elevated blood volume.

Even a small reduction of 8 pounds can bring the blood pressure of obese people with hypertension, to safer levels.

Diabetes

Experts consider obesity to be the primary reason behind insulin resistance which can lead to type 2 diabetes, the most prevalent form of diabetes. **Almost 80% of the people suffering from type 2 diabetes are overweight or obese.** This form of diabetes is developed when the body fails to produce sufficient amounts of insulin, or when the insulin produced is ignored by the body cells.

Obesity has been shown to diminish the ability of insulin to control blood sugar, and the body has to produce greater amounts of insulin in order to regulate the blood sugar. This increases the risk of developing diabetes as the body can fail in effectively controlling the blood sugar.

*Significant weight loss has reversed Type 2 Diabetes
in the majority of obese cases.*

Metabolic Syndrome

Existing metabolic and endocrine disorders are adversely impacted by obesity.

Metabolic syndrome, also known as syndrome X26, affects approximately 20% of overweight people.

It is among the fastest growing health concerns related to obesity in the United States. It is characterized *by a group of health problems*, and these problems amplify the risk of developing fatal health problems.

Osteoarthritis

The joints of the overweight have to bear a lot more pressure due to excess weight, which results in the wearing away of the cartilage tissue that protects them and this increases the risk of developing Osteoarthritis.

Gallbladder Disease

Gallstones are bits of cholesterol that turn into hard rocks in the gallbladder. The risk of developing this condition is higher among the obese, and especially in women.

Cancer

Obesity has been linked to the development of many types of cancers such as gallbladder, kidney, thyroid, pancreas, breast (after menopause) and more.

Sleep Apnea

Obesity often causes sleep apnea, which is a serious breathing disorder that can result in the development of many symptoms that adversely affect health and lifestyle, one of which, is chronic snoring.

Gender Specific Risks

Women

If a woman has a waist size of 35" or more, that means she has a high amount of visceral fat, also known as belly fat. Visceral fat is fat that surrounds your internal organs.
According to the, National Women's Health Resource Center, too much of this type of fat is not a good thing. It is associated with increasing a woman's risk for liver and heart disease.
Fertility can be affected as well in women, where even a 10% body fat loss can increase chances of conception by 25%.

Men

Obese men are more likely to die from prostate cancer, rectum cancer or colon cancer. Sleep apnea is also a serious concern, which, can lead to stroke or heart attack.

Others Ailments And Side Effects

There are many everyday ailments and discomforts that plague the obese, that can and do affect the quality of life. Simply being on one's feet and walking around too much can be an issue because of the chronic knee, joint and foot pain incurred from excess weight.
Lack of energy and the desire to move and play, such as running with kids.

Shortened Life Expectancy

It is also known that obesity shortens life expectancy by 6 years and for the morbidly obese it shortens it by 10.

Emotional Effects

Besides health issues, obesity can also cause emotional, psychological and social wellness issues.

People who are obese are less likely to have a social life. They tend to remain more isolated and are less likely to engage in social activities, mostly due to years of ridicule, stares, laughs and rejection from the opposite sex. That is not the way anyone should live their life. But, the world is a cruel place with a lot of prejudices towards the overweight that can affect personal and work life for the obese.

Many suffer from depression, very low self-esteem and body image disorder. For some, self-loathing becomes a part of everyday life, and causes them to withdraw, which leads to loneliness and a lack of close relationships and romantic involvements.

Children

Almost 3,700 kids and teens under age 20 are diagnosed with Type 2 diabetes each year as a result of obesity.

And, it is projected that by 2050, the number of teen diabetics will increase by nearly 50% to more than 84,000.

45% of children who are diagnosed with type 2 diabetes also have hypertension. Of those, 3% developed kidney disease and 9% of those died from their condition within nine years of the initial diagnosis.

Immediate Effects

According to the Center For Disease Control, children who are obese have high risk factors for high cholesterol and high blood pressure.
A recent study of a sample of 5 to 17 year-olds, showed that 70% had at least one risk factor for cardiovascular disease.
Obese children are more likely to be pre-diabetic and have much higher risks of developing Type 2 diabetes.

Obese kids are also at a higher risk for:

❖ Bone and joint problems
❖ Asthma
❖ Sleep apnea
❖ Low self esteem
❖ Depression
❖ Emotional problems due to teasing

Long Term Effects

Kids who are obese are more likely to be obese as adults, which leads to a lot more health risks and a shorter life expectancy.

Some of the risks include:

❖ Heart disease
❖ Various types of cancers
❖ High blood pressure
❖ Emotional, psychological problems
❖ There is also the lack of energy, and knee and joint pain, that results in limited life activities for those who are extremely obese.

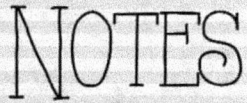

NOTES

Emotional and Psychological Implications

The Social Stigma

There is a huge social stigma and quite a bit of prejudice in the United States towards the overweight. As a society we worship anorexic models, and hot beach bodies, and any shape that strays from that ideal is usually viewed at best in a negative light, and at worst as "disgusting."

For the most part, the overweight and obese are seen as some type of alien creatures that spend their days at fast food drive-thrus ordering piles of food that they will spend the rest of the day gorging on.

As a result of this type of prejudiced thinking, the social relationships and overall connection and belonging in the world is impacted for those who suffer from obesity.

While the world throws judgments and wonders "why don't they just eat less," the overweight know all too well, it is not at all that simple.

Obesity is a Social Problem

Obesity makes people uncomfortable, and when people are uncomfortable, they do not want to be around the person who makes them feel that way. So if you're obese, chances are you're lonely, too, because people simply do not want to be associated with 'the big person.'

This is true for adults as well as children. It's hard to imagine adults being so shallow as to let another person's obesity sway their opinion, but, who said adults always act mature.

Again, the culture that influences the media places a lot of emphasis on youth and beauty, so much so that men and women can feel pressured about how they look, which can perhaps lead to extreme measures that only a mental health practitioner is qualified to address.

Being Labeled

When you're labeled 'fat' that moniker can stay with you throughout your life. Even if you drop some weight you'll still be known to friends and acquaintances who knew you when as 'Fat Lisa' or 'Fat Tom.'
A typical conversation may sound like, 'I wanted to call Lisa,' 'which Lisa "fat" Lisa?' That short but all too telling conversation is a typical one. No one else can see beyond the fact that Lisa is or was fat, regardless that she's accomplished a lot more in her lifetime other than gaining weight. None of that matters however because she is known to her friends, and even family, as 'fat.'
Being fat or to use the more appropriate term 'obese,' is a social problem, a health problem and a psychological problem, which can be just as damaging as the physical and social ones because we live in a society where emphasis has been put on vigor, hot bodies, youth and beauty.
Being fat does not go along with that 'image,' so the 'fat person' is often left out of the 'social circle' simply because he or she is obese.

The Emotional Consequences

The overweight feel the brunt of these attitudes all too well, and the looks, remarks and general stigma can affect their already shaky self-esteem and feelings of self-worth.
Often, this leads to depression, loneliness, isolation and a lack of connection to the world around them.
While this is not always true across the board, for the most part, society's prejudice towards the obese can greatly affect the obese person's ability to belong, and feel worthy of love and attention.

In fact, according to Lancaster General Hospital's Neuropsychology Specialists, 20-70% of obese individuals who are pondering getting bariatric surgery either have a current or a past diagnosis of a psychiatric disorder, with Major Depressive Disorder as the most prominent.

Worse yet is when the overweight's person own family is unsupportive and judgmental with useless statements, such as, "you have to lose weight, stop making excuses," or "it's all in your hands," or "get control of your weight," do nothing more than compound the helplessness and feelings of worthlessness.

For many, romantic relationships can be an uphill struggle as the fear of rejection, which, likely has occurred in the past, can prevent many from reaching out to the opposite sex.

A Vicious Cycle

Often obesity is a vicious cycle.

Society views the obese as weak, and somehow inferior, because they cannot control their weight. The obese who are well aware of this stigma can internalize these judgments, which, puts them at risk for drug and alcohol abuse problems, and mood and anxiety disorders. According to a report by The Medical Clinics of North America, "Psychosocial and behavioral status of patients undergoing bariatric surgery: What to expect before and after surgery," **numerous failed weight loss attempts lead to body image disorders, lowering of an already fragile self-esteem, and a general discomfort of the obese being in their own bodies.**

These feelings lead to further strain on social interactions, personal and romantic relationships with the opposite sex.

Failed weight loss attempts often lead to feelings of helplessness, discouragement, anger, and frustration. Many times this results in the feeling that losing weight will never be a real possibility.

Not surprisingly, a study published in the International Journal of Obesity, showed that of those who lost weight after bariatric surgery, many illustrated major improvements in both their mental and social status and therefore, a much better quality of life.

Children: Teasing And Bullying

For children, being overweight can be especially devastating, and for those who grow into obese adults, those feelings get carried over to adulthood…further aggravating an already vulnerable emotional state. The adult prejudices and overt attitudes towards the overweight is minimal compared to how cruel kids can be.

If adults are uncomfortable around those who are obese and even go as far as to "make fun" of others who are by whispering behind their backs loud enough (so 'Fat Lisa' can hear), imagine what children do to their obese peers.

Children and teens can be extremely cruel, with out loud school hall teasing and name calling that can beseech the obese child. This type of teasing can really a take a toll on their already fragile esteem and self-worth, and lead to serious consequences for their mental and emotional well-being.

This is one of the reasons that it is so important for parents and caregivers to implement a healthy lifestyle and nutritional balance for kids from the start of life. Parents need to educate their children on the health and risk factors and to help them understand portion control and the benefit of a healthy diet.

This would ideally happen before an adolescent's weight is deemed "out of control." Once it's out of control and a child's weight has now been diagnosed as 'obese,' all the health, social and psychological problems that adults face are now the same ones that burden a child. But children lack the maturity or presence of mind in many cases to handle the cruelty of peers.

Let's face it, children can be mean, which, opens up a whole host of problems that the obese child tries to cope with.

Adolescence is difficult enough without the added stress of being 'bullied' by peers simply because of an overweight issue, but, that is the reality.

According to The American Academy of Pediatrics website, **www.healthychildren.org**, the social stigma of childhood obesity can be devastating and lead to serious emotional heartbreak.

In fact, the social stigma, teasing and bullying related to being overweight can cause as much, if not more damage, than the medical repercussions that often accompany obesity.

This teasing causes deep-seated wounds and feelings of shame that usually carry on into adulthood and impact the child's ability to function in a healthy manner in society.

What's the Solution?

First and foremost overweight children need to feel that they can talk honestly about what is going on in school with their parents. Opening lines of communication is the best way to deal with teasing and its consequences.

You can safely assume that if your child is overweight or obese, there has been some type of teasing, it's just human nature.

Children need to know from you, their parent, that the shame is not theirs, and put it where it belongs, on the culprits at school.

Speaking with the school in regards to dealing with rampant teasing is also very important because we have to deal with this issue as a society, as it has become a major problem that has led to teen suicides and can also be sourced in part to the mass amounts of school shootings that have plagued the United States as of late.

Psychotherapy is of course another answer. Another approach, however, is "nipping it in the bud" before psychotherapy becomes necessary.

If a parent sees his or her child's weight begin to spiral out of control that is the time to step in and offer some guidance through education regarding a healthy, low-fat diet and an exercise regimen. It's all about lifestyle changes that will hopefully follow and stay with that child into adulthood.

The same goes for adults whose weight is out of control. Regardless if obesity is a problem at age 21 or 61 or anywhere in between, **it's never too late to incorporate a few lifestyle changes** if the outcome is going to be a healthier and happier new you.

All it takes is a little determination and eventually the weight will come off and best of all stay off because now both the adult and the child have some 'tools' in their arsenal that they can use to combat the urge to 'binge.'

Whatever it takes, there are people who care. And there are people who, if you only ask, will be more than willing to help their obese friend, family member, patient, remain on that train to 'Healthy-Town' through education, encouragement, understanding, compassion and, best of all, love.

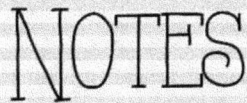

NOTES

Emotional Overeating

Understanding The Problem

Good food is one of the basic pleasures of life. Food is a necessity for all of us. It gives us energy and has an added 'feel good' factor to it as well. Hunger is said to be one of the biggest driving forces in a human being. All that said and done, sometimes we do not know where to stop when it comes to food. It might just be that we enjoy the taste and the flavours of the various delicacies being served and cannot seem to stop even after we are full.

Or might it be something deeper than that?

Nutrition caters to the stomach, but, what of the soul?

Maybe food gives us a kind of solace and company like no other and fills the cravings of the very soul. Emotions are sometimes difficult to understand. But when it comes to food, more and more scientists and researchers and even nutritionists are attributing over eating as an emotional compensation.

This coupled with the growth in various never seen before maladies of the 21st century, like, extremely high levels of stress, loneliness, anxiety, heartbreak, etc. may have turned former healthy eaters, into emotional eaters at some point in time or another.

The classic image in movies and books of a women eating a gallon tub of ice cream after a break up is cliché, but, unfortunately, also reality. Although, as I've mentioned in my FOOD ADDICTION book: **I've witnessed teen boys and adult men consume entire packages of cookies, and cartons of ice cream!**

Cause And Reaction

How often have you felt the need to dig into a pint of ice cream just because you are bored at home and/or are watching television and want to nibble on something?

Or maybe you have this insane urge to have sex and your latest date hasn't called you back and you turn for solace to the chocolate bar lying in the fridge.

Or maybe your boss keeps on asking you to stay after hours and since you are up for promotion, you cannot say 'no'. So you pass those long work hours by with a constant stream of snacks and salty foods.

Maybe nowadays every time you go shopping you end up picking the junk foods and unhealthy convenience foods before you even enter the vegetable section or the fresh food section.

You feel justified in your actions as these foods taste good and make you happy and are always the first things that finish up in your household.

It might also be that such foods are easier to eat as they do not require much [or even no] cooking, and go with your busy schedule and lifestyle.

Whatever the case may be, it seems natural to crave certain foods due to certain reasons at certain points of time in your life.

This is the starting point of emotional eating: where you do not just eat to fill your stomach and satisfy hunger, but, for other reasons.

These are the times that lead to some specific cravings, which, need to be instantly satisfied. But, surprisingly these cravings do not just disappear with the filling of the stomach, but go on and on.

Many are of the opinion that foods cater to a certain vacuum which is momentarily filled with the instant rush that comes with the taste and the psychological satisfaction. The vacuum may be created by financial problems and unemployment which translate to incapability, relationship issues and problems, major fights with loved ones leading to a sense of loneliness and sadness, stress which goes hand in hand with a sense of frustration, health issues and disease, and finally tiredness and fatigue which sometimes means that you feel too lazy to cook or are just happy to eat whatever you have on hand.

Mostly the foods that go hand in hand with such feelings and emotions are fatty foods or junk foods with a high sugar or salt content as they provide an instant burst of energy. In fact, the stress hormone cortisol specifically craves such foods due to the ensuing reaction of pleasure.

Factors of Emotional Eating

There are certain points that can be identified and those that you should know about emotional hunger. With this knowledge you can classify your eating habits better.

1. **Emotional hunger is always sudden.** This is unlike the natural and physical hunger which is a slow and gradual development dealing with speed of digestion and level of exhaustion. Also important to note is the fact that emotional hunger is craving a specific food.

   That means that not just any food can satisfy the need for the moment. A person wants very specific food items when such a hunger pang or desire comes on for example, a bag of salty crisps or a box of chocolate ice cream, or a pizza with extra cheese, the list can go on.

2. Emotional hunger often leads to over eating and/or senseless eating which cannot be stopped. This kind of hunger doesn't connect with whether you are full or not. As mentioned above, this hunger is psychological.

Effects

- This kind of eating habit at one point of time or another can lead to a significant weight gain unless you are blessed with a fantastic metabolism.
- It may also lead to health problems as over eating of fatty foods is extremely unhealthy in the long run.
- Guilt is another by-product of such eating habits. Once the momentary rush of pleasure wears off, one feels incredibly guilty about the food consumed.
- Stomach aches may also follow.
- It might also be that the emotions that triggered the overeating and the hunger do not go away even after you have eaten. This is when you know that you've got to try an alternative to food.

That said, if you have identified the cause of your emotional eating, then address it, instead of keeping it on the back burner.

10 Ways To Overcome Emotional Overeating

❖ Deal with your emotions in positive ways: journaling [I have new journals coming soon to assist you], talking with friends or a therapist, painting, a hobby, go to a movie, anything, but, reaching for the chips and ice cream.

❖ For most people, distraction is a good remedy. Whenever you feel the urge to have a specific food, distract yourself by thinking of something else.

❖ Positive affirmations can help reprogram the mind, and there are plenty available on various topics, or you can write your own.

❖ You could also count till 100 just to give your mind something else to do.

❖ Exercise such as yoga, meditation and other stress-coping skills can help with emotional overeating. Never stop being active. Food needs to be burned, even healthy food and exercise is a known stress reliever. **So take at least 10 minutes out every day (at least) for any physical activity.**

❖ If it is stress, then reduce your work load or sort out the issues that lead to it. Meditation is also wonderful for stress. At Hypnosis Live you can choose a free mp3 **www.hypnosislive.com/choose/a/batlover**

❖ Create rituals. Coping mechanisms in the forms of rituals help to deal with certain triggers, for example, whenever there is the urge to eat because of your emotions, take a bath instead.

❖ If the problem is sadness, then try watching a happy movie or going out with friends or doing something that makes you happy. Whenever I want to be happier *immediately*, I play my favourite music!

❖ Relationship conflicts can be resolved with understanding. If the situation cannot be resolved then get out of it altogether. **Your happiness and peace of mind matters most for the health of your body and soul.**

❖ Also important is to get involved in a healthy activity or to get a hobby. Since emotional eating is psychological, this is a method that works wonders in the long run. For example, join a dance class or take up a course, etc. This will also help you meet new people and provide you with a positive stimulus.

❖ I will post information about these on the Pinterest board I have created for you-so don't forget to check it regularly. In the end, if you love and respect your body, you will respond to these steps and stop the mindless emotional eating, and thus pave the way for a more wholesome and fulfilled life.

❖

The easiest way I have personally found to positively alter my eating habits, and other habits, is to listen to hypnosis

MP3's overnight while I sleep. There are also 'daytime' recordings available. I recommend:
Steve G. Jones
Tellman Knudsen (The New Hypnotists)
Hypnosis Live

They have all sorts of MP3's that can help you relax, increase confidence, reduce stress, lose weight, exercise more,etc..

- *See my Pinterest board pin for more help:*
  www.pinterest.com/petralovesbats/childhood-obesity

NOTES

Weight Loss Options For Obese Adults

It is true that the obese process food differently than those who are not, not only physically and internally, but, also psychologically.

More likely than not you have dieted your whole life; one diet after another, losing, gaining, losing, gaining on an endless yo-yo cycle. This is because diets don't work, they are temporary, hence the reference, "getting on a diet" and "getting off a diet".

Instead, consider lifestyle changes and changing eating tastes and habits.

> *The most important element of successful long term weight management is an inherent change in lifestyle habits, versus the "diet mindset", which is a short term solution where people get "on" and "off".*

For example, people who quit eating sugar, often remark that when they do occasionally bite on something sweet, like a cookie or donut, the sugar is intolerable and they cannot finish it. That is because they have permanently altered their taste for it.

That is a permanent lifestyle change.

Ordering all burger combos with a side salad instead of fries, without even thinking about it at the drive thru. And with iced water rather than soda pop.

That is a permanent lifestyle change.

Choosing water or plain tea as a drink with lunch, without ever considering full sugar soda.

That is a permanent lifestyle change.

Regularly reaching for a side of vegetables, instead of mashed potatoes and gravy.

That is a permanent lifestyle change.

Serving yourself one tablespoon of mashed potatoes, versus 3 or 4 each time you swallow.

That is a permanent lifestyle change.

Consistently getting regular exercise.

That is a permanent lifestyle change.

Consistent exercise, portion control and burning more calories than you eat is at the center of healthy weight management.

Changing the mindset and tastes can go a long way to begin the road to fitness, this is why it is critical to consider weight loss methods carefully. In the past few decades, there has been an explosion in the number of weight loss plans. Some of them are effective, some of them are not so effective, and there are some plans so outrageously extreme, that a person would probably be better off obese than following them.

The key to finding the best method of permanent weight loss is any plan that focuses on making permanent and lasting eating and fitness lifestyle changes.

Lifestyle Changing Weight Loss Options

Behaviour Modification

The National Heart Lung and Blood Institute points out that there are various triggers that cause people to over eat.

For example, while watching TV, or during stress, or when going out with certain friends.

Identifying and changing such habits can be really helpful in weight control.

Be conscious of what you eat and why. Stay aware of your bad habits and work on changing them. Many people eat not because they are hungry, but, for other reasons.

Monitor portion sizes, and eat healthy foods. Seek professional help to analyze and become aware of the psychology behind your eating habits.

Registered Dietician/Nutritionist

Seeking the services of a registered dietician/nutritionist is a great way to form a weight loss plan that will be customized just for you to yield the best results.
This is covered by most insurance plans and is required as the first step in the approval process for bariatric surgery by most insurance companies.
A good registered dietician or nutritionist will have sufficient knowledge regarding the latest developments and research findings, along with in-depth understanding of the human body.

They will adjust the program according to your needs and your food preferences.

This becomes especially important if you have conditions such as high blood pressure, high cholesterol, cancer or diabetes.

The dietician/nutritionist will educate you about the food choices that you need to make, and the correct daily calorie intake, in order to lose weight and improve your health.

Another big benefit of seeing a nutritionist is the fact that **regular appointments and weigh-ins make you accountable to someone other than yourself, and this can be a good motivator and facilitator of staying on track.**

Consulting A Doctor

Consulting a doctor for weight loss offers similar benefits as consulting a registered nutritionist/dietician. They can keep a regular check on your health and monitor your progress accordingly. They can also order lab tests to check various parameters regarding the body's status, or health conditions that might have developed as a result of obesity.

Doctors also have various medical treatments that they can prescribe as needed. For some a short term treatment can include diet pills and also there are various bariatric surgery options for weight loss that are used for the morbidly obese.

Those who are pre-diabetic and have high insulin numbers can ask their doctor about a medication called Metformin, which, helps to stave off diabetes, lower the impact of insulin trigger foods and really helps with weight loss.

Weight Watchers

How to separate the better diet plans from the rest? Check whether they focus on changing your lifestyle for a gradual weight loss that can be maintained for years.

Weight loss will not lead to a healthier life by following plans that emphasize drastic reduction of calories to achieve it. You will be trading one set of problems with another. Follow plans that promote the formation of better habits.

Weight Watchers is one such plan. It emphasizes on motivating followers to change their eating, cooking, grocery shopping and dining habits for a healthier lifestyle, along with motivating them to exercise too.

Its effectiveness has been proven by studies that showed that participants of the Weight Watchers plan had significantly more weight loss than the self-help soldiers.

Although, there is nothing wrong with soldiering on your own. It is all about healthy habits. The internet is filled with knowledge, and an effective weight loss plan can be formed by filtering the reliable content. For those who cannot do that, Weight Watchers is a good option.

Costs

They will charge you for their services. For your money you can attend optional group meetings for support, use their app to chart your progress, access the online community and their website, which offers a good collection of recipes, tips and useful tools.

The plan uses a point-based system to measure progress.

Each food item is assigned a point based on their nutritional content.

A daily point allowance is assigned to individuals based on different parameters.

A great option, if you can afford to pay their fees, which, really are minimal.

The Atkins Diet

The Atkins diet is a popular low-carbohydrate lifestyle change diet, which has shown to be effective in promoting weight loss and improving health for thousands of people around the world.

In this diet, cutting back on high carbohydrate foods, such as rice, bread, pasta and sugary foods is required, and when they say cut back, they really mean it.

Coincidentally this is the exact eating plan prescribed to those who have Type 2 Diabetes or are in a pre-diabetic state, which is mostly tied to obesity, so it may be the ideal solution for that group.

Any Negatives?

Studies have not demonstrated any major risks with the long-term adoption of such a diet. In fact, they have demonstrated that such diets can possibly benefit people with conditions such as cancer, type-2 diabetes and epilepsy, and improve cholesterol levels. However, people with severe kidney disease are recommended to avoid Atkins diet. Always check with your doctor before starting this or any other weight loss plan.

The Atkins Stages

Atkins is a low carb diet plan. It allows for very few carbs daily initially, and then gradually some carbs are re-introduced.

The diet consists of stages, the first of which is called Induction, where a drastic cut in carbohydrate intake induces the body into a state, known as, Ketosis, where the body burns existing fat instead of ingested carbs for energy.

The Induction Stage

Limit daily carbohydrate intake to 20 grams, and those are limited to certain vegetables.

Grains, such as rice, bread, and pasta, have to be cut out from the diet, along with starchy vegetables [peas, potatoes] and dairy products other than cream, cheese and butter.

No legumes, nuts or seeds.

Absolutely no sugar, including refined and that from foods like fruit.
- Alcohol and caffeine are banned too.

Consequent Stages

In the ongoing weight loss stages, more vegetables, legumes, seeds, nuts, whole grains, and berries and other fruit can be added to the diet. Considering the major changes that need to be made and drastic limitation of food choices in the first stage, this diet may not be ideal for everyone, but nonetheless, it is an effective one.

The diet also recommends 30 minutes of almost daily exercise. The more exercise one gets, the more carbs are allowed to be eaten daily.

Vegetarians who follow the diet start in the second phase, as following the first stage is not possible without meat, fish and poultry. The diet is extremely challenging to follow for vegans, but, not impossible.

Success Rates

Success rates with Atkins for those who follow it are really high. Many lose 10, 15 or more pounds in the Induction stage and continue to lose until they reach their goals.

This is a lifestyle changing plan, as it teaches you to choose healthy foods and regulates blood sugars which eliminates rampant cravings. Many report great results.

Costs

There are no fees for this diet, all the details can be accessed for free at their website.

Support

Online forums, groups, meals plans and some helpful tools are present on the official Atkins website. Overall, the Atkins diet is an option that will be an effective weight loss plan for people with strong determination. For others, adhering to the rules and limitations might be challenging.

Medifast

Medifast's weight loss program is a medical diet, created by a doctor and is based on meal replacements. The "Medifast 5 & 1 Plan" allows the participants to enjoy six meals a day. However, five of those will be replacements meals offered by Medifast.

Typically, participants lose about 1 or 2 pounds each week on this plan. Once the desired weight target is achieved, calories are gradually added over a period of 6 weeks.

Medifast recommends following their "3 & 3 plan," three meal replacements with three meals, to keep the weight off indefinitely.

There are about 70 meal replacements offered by Medifast. The participant's own meal must contain a good quantity of lean protein, three vegetable servings and a maximum of two servings of healthy fats. Sauces, condiments, dressing and a single snack each day, such as Jell-O, a Popsicle, celery, gum, or some almonds, pistachios or walnuts, are also allowed.

Everything that is not included in the food list approved by Medifast is off limits, and the list doesn't include alcohol and dairy products.

Optional in-person meetings are offered at Medifast Weight Control Centers. There are about 100 such centers across US. The program encourages participants to exercise, but specific workout programs are not offered.

Costs

Seems like a decent choice, but there are caveats. Participants have reported that the meal replacements are not that palatable. Then there is the cost factor. Those meal replacements don't come for free.

As of June 2014, a 4-week package with 140 servings costs $339.00USD. Hence, the program might not be fit for those who don't wish to spend so much.

However, for those who lack motivation and want an easy plan that guarantees some weight loss when followed properly and can afford to pay the costs, Medifast is a solid option.

It also has replacements that fit the needs of different specialized diet groups, such as vegetarians, vegans, gluten free and low salt.

Jillian Michaels Fitness and Weight Loss Program

Jillian Michaels is a world renowned fitness expert who is one of the stars of the hit TV reality show, the Biggest Loser. She has helped transform many bodies from obesity to complete fitness.

She offers a structured online weight loss and fitness program whose goal is to provide long term solutions to healthy weight management, with a strong emphasis on healthy eating and exercise.

Membership includes a complete diet and exercise plan that is geared towards individual needs.

Each plan is designed based on:

❖ Current weight

❖ Eating habits

❖ Level of exercise activity

The Jillian Michaels Weight Loss Approach

The program determines the precise amount of calories one needs to lose weight each week.

Members are taught to make healthy choices, learn about the best foods and also various healthy cooking methods.

The exercise portion of the plan designs a custom workout program for each member that is based on their weight, height and general fitness level.

Everything is done online, and there is a strong online support system.

Benefits

- ❖ Custom tailored for individual needs.
- ❖ Not a temporary diet, but, a complete lifestyle change program that incorporates food and fitness.
- ❖ Sets goals with detailed action steps to achieve those.
- ❖ Food and exercise plans are provided each week.
- ❖ Learning to change your life is made easy with detailed information about which foods to eat and why, and also which exercises to do, and the parts of the body they work.
- ❖ All workouts can be done at home.
- ❖ Support from other members through an active online forum.
- ❖ Meal delivery is offered, for those that don't want to cook.
- ❖ Many real people testimonials of success.
- ❖ When followed as recommended this program will without a doubt result in weight loss, even for those that need to lose 50 or 100 pounds.

Costs

There is a fee for the program, but, it is very reasonable.

NHS Weight Loss Plan

UK's National Health Service offers a 12-week plan for losing weight, completely free of cost. No wonder it was voted as the best healthcare system among 11 developed countries in a report by the Commonwealth Fund, a foundation based in Washington, USA. So is it the holy grail of weight loss plans?

Not completely, but that is not because of any fault in the plan itself. The reason behind that is that the plan focuses on healthy and gradual weight loss by encouraging the participants to change their lifestyle, which is exactly what some people don't want to pursue. They want quick fixes that the program doesn't offer.

What does the program offer?

It offers tips to help you weed out the stuff and habits that lead to obesity, and provides valuable information and support to shed the pounds gradually, and then maintain a healthy lifestyle for life.

You can download the 12-week guide, which offers weekly progression tips to lose weight over a period of 12 weeks and transition smoothly into better habits, without any cost from their website.

A weekly chart is also provided that you can print and use to check your progress. It also promotes exercise and provides tips to adopt a more active lifestyle.

A nine week guide which helps people transition from a couch potato to someone who can run 5k is also provided. There's also a weight loss forum and an email support service.

Overall, it's a good, sensible weight loss plan with adequate support service.

The best part, it doesn't cost a penny.

Overeaters Anonymous 12 Step Program

The focus of Overeaters Anonymous is not on being a club for dieting and calorie counting. They focus on the underlying issues that lead to obesity.

There are no specific guidelines according to which members are incorporated in the group. Anyone having problems related to compulsive eating or with food addiction or any type of dysfunction associated with food can join the group for support.

Therefore, even though it is not a weight loss plan in itself, the positivity that will develop with support techniques will help those who find it difficult to stick with diets and hence, prevent their weight from increasing, or even decrease it.

Bariatric Surgery Options To Treat Morbid Obesity

Bariatric surgery is the term used for all procedures that are performed surgically for treating morbid obesity.

The size of the stomach is reduced with a gastric band, or by removing a portion of the stomach, or by re-routing and resectioning the small intestines (gastric bypass surgery).

Long term studies have shown effectiveness of the procedures in significantly reducing the weight and helping the patients recover from diabetes, along with improving their risk factors of cardiovascular diseases and reducing mortality rates. However, compared with usual care, no survival benefits were found among older and severely obese patients by a study conducted on Veteran Affairs patients.

Types Of Surgery

Surgical procedures of two types are employed:

- Malabsorptive procedures- These procedures block the normal absorption of nutrients by diverting the food from the stomach. It is sent to a lower part of the digestive tract where the digestive juices cannot mix properly with the food.
- Restrictive procedures- These procedures decrease the intake of food by restricting the size of the stomach.

Both of these procedures can be combined together in weight loss surgery.

1. **Roux-en-Y Gastric Bypass (RYGBP)**

   In RYGBP the weight loss is achieved by malabsorption and gastric restriction. The patient can feel satiated even after small meals if the stomach size is reduced to a small gastric pouch of 30cc. The duodenum is bypassed by connecting the small pouch to a segment of jejunum, and thus, reducing the absorption of nutrients. RYGBP procedures can be laparoscopic or open.

2. **Biliopancreatic Diversion with Duodenal Switch (BPD/DS)**

   BPD/DS procedures also use malabsorption and gastric restriction to achieve weight loss. However, when compared to RYGBP, the size of the partially resected stomach is more generous. The intake is not reduced dramatically, and the patients can have relatively normal sized portions while still reducing weight as substantial malabsorption is achieved by bypassing the duodenum and jejunum. BPD/DS procedures can also be laparoscopic or open.

3. **Adjustable Gastric Banding (AGB)**

   Only gastric restriction is used to achieve weight loss in AGB procedures. A gastric pouch band with a small capacity of about 15 to 30cc's is created which encircles the stomach's upper portions. AGB procedures allow the size of the gastric pouch to be modified when required, as the bands are adjustable. The size is changed depending on the rate of the patient's weight loss. AGB is a laparoscopic surgical procedure.

4. Sleeve Gastrectomy

In sleeve gastrectomy, the volume of the stomach is reduced while maintaining the continuity of the lesser curvature of the stomach as sleeve gastrectomy is majorly a gastrectomy of the greater curvature. Earlier, sleeve gastrectomy formed the first step of a two-step procedure while performing the RYGBP, but in recent times it has been offered and performed as a stand-alone surgery.

5. Vertical Gastric Banding (VGB)

Similar to AGB, weight loss is achieved by gastric restriction in VGB procedures. A narrow pouch or inlet is created by stapling the upper portions of the stomach. The pouch or inlet remains connected with the rest of the stomach.

To prevent the enlargement of the opening in the future, a small band which cannot be adjusted is also placed around the new inlet. In this procedure the weight loss results solely from the eating of smaller portions by the patients as the feeling of satiety is experienced quickly. **VGB procedures and not performed any longer.**

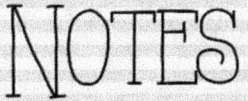

NOTES

Exercise Options For The Obese

Control your diet and exercise, and you'll soon see the results. It sounds easy, and it might be easy for some. However, a lot people who are battling with obesity and want to lose weight find initiating the exercise part tough, especially when they haven't worked out much, or at all, in their entire life.

And for some, it is just not possible to move well, due to extreme excess weight or a very long term sedentary lifestyle. In such cases it becomes extremely important to start slowly and comfortably.

Someone might approach the initial stages with a lot of enthusiasm and gusto, only to find that their body aches and pains in ways that can be a real deterrent to continuing. That might put them off from exercise for a long time and lead to a negative state of mind.

Another real issue for those who are extremely heavy is that moving may just be difficult, if not, impossible. Knee, joint and foot pain are all concerns.

So what is the ideal way to proceed? The answer is simple: slow and easy.

If you are obese, your joints are carrying a lot of extra weight, and your bones might be brittle too. You can easily stress them, which can cause several short and long-term injuries.

Similarly, there might be misalignments and muscular imbalances in the body structure because of a highly sedentary lifestyle. This means that muscles need to work harder in order to keep the structure stable. This is even more dangerous when those muscles are not used to working at all! Many people also have a reduced range of motion of joints, making some activities tougher for them.

Seeking professional help is one answer, and also here are the best exercise options for a controlled yet effective start of the new phase of your life:

Personal Trainer

Any decent personal trainer will know how to progress carefully. They will form an exercise regimen according to your limitations and capabilities, and guide you constantly in the right direction.

Your local YMCA might be a good option too, and they offer lower cost options.
Taking a friend along will help you if you're shy. Working out with a friend is a lot more fun. They will provide motivation, and some healthy competition won't hurt either.

Walking

Too broke for a personal trainer?
Don't worry; we have just scratched the surface. Walking is a completely free and potentially fun exercise. Head out to your neighborhood park, street or anywhere you like.
Feel free to explore the city or your favorite wall on the treadmill.
Many prefer the outdoors, but, everyone has his or her own preferences. Some walls are extremely interesting.
Walking is a low impact and simple exercise. Just make sure that you walk as briskly as you can. No need to rush, all you have to do is to ensure that it is a walk and not a stroll. Start with a time limit at which you are comfortable, and slowly increase it. An increment of 10 or more minutes every week will work.

Once you can walk comfortably for 30 minutes continuously, start increasing your pace a bit. A walk every alternate day initially will be ideal. Later on as you become more proficient at this wonderful skill, you can walk 5 days a week. Keep yourself hydrated and remember, no snacks from the hot dog stand.

Swimming/Water Aerobics

Swimming can be perfect for those who are willing to learn the skill as it works all parts of the body and doesn't put any strain on the joints. Joining a swimming class would be the ideal way to start.
Although, if you don't want to devote time and pick up a new, potentially challenging skill, there is another alternative that works well too: water aerobics.
The buoyant force of the water reduces the stress on your joints and makes the movements easier to perform, and the water itself resists the movements, making water aerobics an effective workout routine.
Many places also offer water yoga classes. They can help you gain flexibility quicker if you find performing yoga poses extremely challenging.

Portable Peddler

A great piece of fitness equipment is the Portable Peddler. This machine can be used while sitting down and can be done from anywhere. Peddle for 7 minutes, rest for 5, and then peddle again. Increase time as fitness levels increase.

Yoga/Pilates

Yoga and Pilates are body-conditioning programs known worldwide for their effectiveness.

Not only will they help you burn calories, they will also increase your range of motion and correct body alignment, making you more comfortable with your body. However, don't expect results in a week. Your body will take time to shirk off the sedentary habits reinforced with years of practicing.

It is also because of that sedentary habit that you should start with an experienced trainer. Many of your skills, such as proprioception (awareness regarding the position of body in the space), flexibility, strength and endurance might be below average.

A trainer will ensure that you don't injure yourself right at the beginning of your new lifestyle. Proper alignment and form is very important in both yoga and Pilates. Thankfully, all good instructors pay a lot of attention to these in their classes.

Again, if you are broke or/and have confidence in your ability to follow the instructions properly and not injure yourself, you can consider buying a good yoga/Pilates training video.

Read reviews online before buying so that you know what you are getting. Make sure you buy the basic one for beginners; too much confidence might be counterproductive. You can also find workout videos that are made especially for big folks with limited flexibility.

Exercise Bikes

Biking is also a low impact activity that won't be harsh on your joints. However, riding a real bike requires balance and some basic training, and a few falls while training are inevitable. That might be problematic for some people as their hands and wrists might not be able to support the extra body weight, ending the fun activity in the emergency room. However, smart humans have invented this machine known as a stationary bike, no balancing required! Just sit and peddle.

Riding a stationary bike is a great way to start burning calories. Go slow at first and then progress as you get more fit and build endurance.

You can find many different types of stationary bikes on the market. Some of them might not be comfortable for everyone because of the tiny seats, but many models have padded chairs with a backrest, which would be ideal for those who are extremely obese as it will prevent back pain too.

Elliptical Trainers

Then there are elliptical machines. The machine offers the same movement patterns as jogging without any of the stress caused by the striking of the foot on the ground. This is extremely important as some people who are transitioning from a sedentary lifestyle might have brittle bones.

If you don't have space at your home to keep one, or if it is out of your budget, you can head to any gym. Most gyms keep a couple of elliptical trainers handy at least as they are popular, and their popularity is well justified. They form a safe and an extremely effective method of cardio training.

Recumbent Elliptical Machine

Another great method of exercise for those that have a hard time moving and walking. This one offers a complete elliptical cardio workout while sitting. These machines offer a full body workout that works the arms and legs and increases heart rate for fat burning with the low impact of sitting.

Workouts From The Couch

For those who really have a hard time moving due to extreme obesity or just to add more exercise while watching TV, several workouts can be done from the couch.

First, getting some lightweight free weights and doing bicep curls is a great way to get the blood pumping.

Another option is leg lifts that can be done while laying on your side on the floor, or by simply lifting your legs in front of you while sitting on the couch.

NOTES

Obesity In Children

1 out of every 10 children in the UK and 1 out of every 5 children in the US are hugely overweight.

This is not just a problem for these two nations, but, a malaise threatening the entire world, though the US has the highest numbers. In a dichotomous scenario where thousands of children from many developing nations or poor families struggle to get even one square meal a day, many children from affluent homes or developed nations are turning obese due to an excess of food and a lack of exercise.

This phenomenon has been further fueled by a development in technology with video games replacing outdoor play and family walks and trips cut short or substituted with television time.

Also on the rise is the busy fast paced life wherein parents are working or children have excessively packed schedules with school, practice classes, coaching, etc. This has led to a lack of time to prepare wholesome healthy foods and instead has created a growing dependence on packaged meals.

With everything available around the clock and easily delivered and a growth in fast food joints and restaurants at an easy accessible distance, eating out or grabbing 'fast' food is the norm rather than an exception. With all this going on, children are also more attuned to junk food, as fried food seems tastier than having vegetables, and candy tastes better than fruit.

Childhood obesity does not differ from adult obesity. Just like their adult counterparts, children will accumulate fat cells on their body if they consume more calories than their body burns off. A pattern that can lead to obesity if it is not corrected in time, and statistics show that it is not being checked.

In fact, childhood obesity has tripled since the 1970s and it seems the "Super Size" world has finally caught up with us.

Top Causes/Risk Factors of Childhood Obesity

Rates of obesity have grown alarmingly in the age group of 6-19 years in the past few decades.
What is the reason behind this increase?
Actually, no single cause or factor can be blamed for obesity. It is a complex problem, and often there are multiple factors working simultaneously. Following are some of the top causes of childhood obesity:

Poor Diet

Poor choices when it comes to eating are a major factor behind the rise of obesity, both in adults and children. **Foods that are high in sugar**, such as candies, chips, cookies and other baked desserts, soft drinks and other items sold at the vending machine, **along with foods that are high in fats and sodium**, such as fast foods, provide many calories without offering much nutrition. Consumption of these foods has grown over the years.

These often serve as snack options, but what people don't realize is that these foods are usually calorie-dense and often provide more calories when combined than a main course meal.

Research has shown that kids in America are now getting, as much as, 27% of their daily calories from such snacks. This problem is often worsened by the fact that many kids don't get a healthy lunch either. Convenient options for lunch, which can be packed easily and often come from pre-packaged food items, are to be blamed in several cases. **Processed foods have replaced home-cooked, healthy meals. They also promote overeating.**

Tantalizing commercials that are on air every day, large sizes of portions and lack of dietary fiber, thereby reducing satiety, are to be blamed for tempting kids, and adults too, into consuming these foods more often. Sure enough, **research has shown that sugar and fast food can be as addictive as some drugs.**

When your kitchen cabinets are filled with junk food, those are the only choices you provide your kids.

Lack Of Physical Activity

In the modern era, where so many things are easier for us because of technological advancement, a sedentary lifestyle has become a major problem. It is also a major cause of childhood obesity.

Using cars to travel to school and short distances; overprotecting kids from the dangers of outdoor play activities; and television, computers and gaming consoles have made the lifestyle of kids extremely sedentary.

Many kids lack sufficient physical activity at the preschool age itself, which makes it less probable that these kids will adopt a more active lifestyle in the future. Not only do these kids miss the benefits of regular exercise, the lifestyle they adopt comes with numerous health negatives.

Experts recommended that kids get 60 minutes of moderate physical activity every day.

It doesn't have to be all at once, 2 or 3 sessions of 20-30 minutes each, works too.

Parents should promote activities such as dancing, biking, dodge ball, tag, walking, running, various sports and activities that require physical movement.

Improper Environment

Yes, global warming and steadily reducing forest cover are a reality, and scary ones too, but they are not the environmental concerns that cause childhood obesity. **"Improper environment" refers to the conditions kids encounter at home and at school.**

If parents don't set an example and adopt a healthier lifestyle themselves, the odds of kids doing so decreases.

Kids should not be blamed for their addiction to processed and high sugar foods if all they find upon opening the kitchen cabinets and the refrigerator are chocolates, cookies, ice cream, crackers and readymade processed and canned foods.

Keeping your refrigerator and cabinets stocked with healthier food options, such as vegetables, fruits and nuts, will ensure that kids eat healthy food. Of course, this doesn't mean that you should cut the "bad" food items completely.

A treat once a week doesn't hurt. Much. However, a treat every day hurts a lot.

Similarly, kids will sit and watch television for hours if they see that that is what their parents do every day. It is important to instill healthier habits into your lifestyle, so that your kids can learn by example.

Unfortunately, obese parents can pass their unhealthy habits to their kids, and so those children are more at risk due to genetics and environment. The nature and nurture factors can combust here with disastrous results for the kids.

Schools too need to focus on providing proper information regarding the consequences of being overweight, and help kids avoid or overcome these conditions.

Socio-Economic Factors

Obesity rates are at 30.4% for preschoolers in low income households. This is due to the fact that **unhealthy foods are cheap, including, frozen foods, crackers and cookies that are high in calories and low in nutritional value.**
They are easy to get and cheaper than fresh healthy options. There is also the fact that there is less access to safe recreational areas for kids to play and run in low income areas.

Other Causes

In addition to the above mentioned major causes, there are a few more factors that can exacerbate or lead to obesity. Some of these factors can also be the major factor in some cases.

- **Genetics** - Genes can also play a part in childhood obesity. Some kids might have inherited genes from their parents that make them susceptible to gaining weight easily. These genes might have been useful in the past, when food was scarce and people had a much more active lifestyle, but in the modern era, these genes can be problematic, especially with reduced physical activity. In a few rare cases, obesity can be linked to genetic conditions like Prader Willi syndrome.

- **Medical conditions** - There are a few medical conditions that can lead to obesity: hypothyroidism, growth hormone deficiency and Cushing's syndrome. Eating disorders, such as night eating syndrome and binge eating disorder, can also be a factor in some cases.

- **Psychological factors** - Food can also serve as a coping mechanism. A kid can turn to eating high-sugar and high-fat foods, **which are recognized as rewards by the brain**, in negative situations to cope with the intense emotions. Loneliness, death or a divorce in the family, bullying, abuse, anxiety and boredom are a few examples of issues that can lead to binge eating for coping.

- **Medications-** Some medications prescribed to teens and kids can also cause weight gain as a side effect, these include:
    - Mirtazapine, Imipramine. Paroxetine and other antidepressants
    - Anticonvulsants, especially Gabapentin, Vigabartin and Sodium Valproate
    - Antipsychotics such as Aripiprazole, Clozapine, Chlorpromazine, Olanzapine, Quetiapine, Pimozide, Quetiapine, and Risperidone
    - Corticosteroids

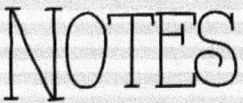

NOTES

What Parents Can Do To Prevent Obesity

Who wants to deny their children food? The problem, however, if left to their own devices many children would eat cupcakes for dinner and popcorn for dessert rather than a well-balanced, nutritious meal. Perhaps one of the greatest hardships a parent has to go through during their child's adolescence is having to persistently say, "No."

It's little wonder that 'No' is usually the first word repeated next to 'mama' or 'dada' in junior's new but growing vocabulary. But, as children and parents grow older and arguments ensue, which, unfortunately takes its toll on both child and parent, parents sometimes give in to the pressure.

Before that scenario becomes reality, however, providing smart nutrition and being involved in how much physical activity kids get is up to the parents.

If not, any child is at risk to become a part of the growing obesity numbers in the under 20 population and just another statistic. And, those kids that are prone to weight gain may spiral out of control if not for the discipline displayed by the parents. It's all too common that after a while of 'giving in,' the 'chubby' cute kid can quickly turn into a fat one on the precipice of obesity, which is a harsh reality for parents as well as their children.

Knowledge Is Key

The first thing parents need to do is to educate themselves on what it means to live a healthy lifestyle in terms of weight management and fitness.

It is crucial to understand:
Healthy Diet
Proper Nutrition
How much from each food group a child should eat
Portion control and calorie requirements for each age group and sex of the child.
Importance and application of regular physical activity for kids.
This kind of knowledge is absolutely necessary in order to instill healthy habits in kids that will prevent obesity and stick with them into adulthood to facilitate life-long healthy lifestyles.

Teach By Example

Children are impressionable. As parents, you see in your children their adoration for a superhero or the latest 'pop-tart' who churns out silly pop tunes for their admiring young fans. What you didn't see coming however is your ten, eleven, twelve-year-old being the butt of jokes and ridicule because of obesity.

You may ask yourself 'how did this happen?' That is usually the time when you have to take a long hard look at **your lifestyle**. Were you, as a parent, doing all you could to help your impressionable prepubescent teen navigate the waters? It's not a secret.

> Children look up to their mother and father, which is a big responsibility for any parent, but as big as that responsibility is, it's the parents' obligation to do all they can to set the right example.

Unfortunately, many adults who have children do not realize that their habits, both good and bad, impact their child's early years, which is why it is imperative as a parent to be the model of decorum.

If your child sits down with a bowl of ice cream every night because that's what dad does, perhaps the time has come for dad to grab an apple or a pear instead, which will hopefully encourage the impressionable child to do the same.

Exercise is another area where parents can teach by example. If weekends are spent laying on the couch in front of the television, likely that is the same thing the kids will be doing.

But, if each weekend the parents are out at the park, playing tennis, walking on the beach, or playing basketball at the driveway net, then that is where the kids will be as well.

Provide A Healthy Diet From The Start

It makes sense to begin introducing vitamin and protein rich food into your child's diet early, but like anything else, in moderation.

An infant does not yet have the inherent tools to say 'enough' and will continue to eat, if the parents let him or her do so.

It is therefore good parenting to start introducing into your youngster's diet fruits, vegetables and lean cuts of meat that will provide all the nutrients needed for a healthy well-balanced diet.

Again, moderation is also a factor. Just because your three-year-old loves bacon doesn't mean you should let the child eat an entire pound.

The Food Groups

- Grains
- Fruits
- Low or non-fat dairy
- Vegetables
- Lean Protein

The portions and daily servings depend on the age and sex of the child.

Sugar Fat and Salt

Sugar, fat and salt should be consumed in moderation.

The American Heart Association recommends that kids older than 2 should get about 30% of their daily calories from fat.

Of that, only 7% to 10% should come from saturated fats. Trans fats should be avoided altogether.

They also recommend that kids consume no more than 12 grams or three teaspoons of sugar per day.

Recommended Salt Intake for Kids

❖ 1,500 mg per day for kids 1 to 3 years old

❖ 1,900 mg per day for kids 4 to 8 years old

❖ 2,200 mg per day for kids 9 to 13 years old

The Not So Happy " Happy Meal"

A McDonalds Cheeseburger Happy Meal has:

670 Calories

46 Grams Fat

7.5 Saturated Fat

28 Grams Sugar

840mg Sodium

That is a lot of calories, fat, sugar and sodium from just one meal!

Especially when you consider the fact that for kids, ages 4 to 8, the recommended daily caloric intake is between 1200 to 2000 calories max, 1900mg max for sodium, a max of 12 grams for sugar, and saturated fat should be less than 1% of daily calories.

AND

Most of the foods included in the Happy Meal, have little or NO nutritional value.

Should you never buy Happy Meals for your kids?

Maybe; that is a decision parents need to make. There are many super active kids who can easily handle the occasional treat of the Happy Meal.

The decision really depends on goals beyond that in preventing obesity, such as, heart healthy eating habits they will take with them into adulthood.

Should happy meals be nightly dinner?

Probably not.

Healthier Options For Happy Meals:
Order apple slices instead of fries with the meal.
Swap the Coke for water or whole milk.

Healthy Cooking

Healthy cooking, such as, steamed vegetables and fruit smoothies are a great way to introduce to your children heart-healthy foods at an early age.

If broccoli or cauliflower is met with disdain, try pouring a little cheese sauce onto the vegetables.

If you as a parent, start when your children are young and give them a lot of fruits and vegetables, as they get older they will naturally gravitate toward those foods.

Engaging kids by allowing them to assist in cooking and meal preparation as appropriate for their age will greatly increase the chances of their interest in any types of food they helped prepare. They can be asked to help with all types of cooking and baking. Kids love to help, it will teach them how to cook healthy and will make them proud and filled with a sense of accomplishment.

Provide Healthy Snacks

What's inside your cupboards and refrigerator says a lot about your diet.

Keeping healthy food in the home is the first and maybe most important step in dictating what your child will eat.

This may be easier said than done, but, it is just a fact of raising healthy and fit kids.

It's not difficult, but, it does take a conscious effort to keep wholesome snacks in the refrigerator so the first thing your child reaches for are the celery sticks with peanut butter or the chopped carrot sticks.

It's up to parents to introduce early in a child's life
the world of fruits and vegetables as wholesome snacking.

Even baked goods such as oatmeal raisin cookies can be made without processed sugar. Simply cut back on the sugar or use a sugar substitute, like Applesauce. Add shredded carrot, or zucchini into the mix.

Be creative.
If your child naturally reaches for a handful of Oreos after school, he or she is probably craving fat.

Fat however is loaded with vitamin E, certainly an essential vitamin, so instead of Oreo cookies introduce early in life foods that are naturally rich in vitamin E such as avocado or nuts.

Get creative and turn the avocados into a delicious guacamole dip with baked pita chips for dipping or keep Nutella on hand, a delicious hazelnut spread that can be put on whole grain breads, crackers and waffles.

There are many ways to replace unhealthy snacks.
All it takes is a little imagination and an extra half an hour in the kitchen before your child flies into the house and goes right for the cupboard or refrigerator looking for something to eat.
Instead, have it ready or have it already made in the refrigerator, this makes it more likely that that is what they will eat.

List Of Healthy Snacks Ideas

- ❖ String Cheese
- ❖ Fresh fruit
- ❖ Whole grain crackers
- ❖ Low fat frozen yogurt
- ❖ Sorbet
- ❖ Trail mixes with dried fruit and nuts
- ❖ Fresh fruit smoothies
- ❖ All fruit popsicles
- ❖ Frozen bananas
- ❖ Homemade frozen berry pops
- ❖ Apples with almond or peanut butter
- ❖ Applesauce
- ❖ Graham crackers
- ❖ Fig bars
- ❖ Vanilla wafers
- ❖ Fruit with caramel dip
- ❖ Kashi GoLean bars
- ❖ Granola (check labels to verify sugar content)
- ❖ Baked chips
- ❖ Vegetable chips
- ❖ Soy crisps
- ❖ Rice cakes
- ❖ Unbuttered popcorn
- ❖ Pita chips
- ❖ Whole wheat pretzels

- ❖ Nuts
- ❖ Raisins
- ❖ Dried cherries
- ❖ Fruit leather
- ❖ Cereal bars
- ❖ Banana chips
- ❖ Low or zero sugar nutrition bars

Limit Sugary Foods

Clean out the refrigerator and the cupboards of any and all food that are unhealthy and replace them with fruits, vegetables and healthy sweets. Become more creative in the kitchen and soon you are bound to see some changes both in your children's attitude and in a shrinking waistline.

Healthier Baked Goods

Learn how to make healthier baked goods.
There are plenty of substitutions that can be used to create tasty sweets that are lower in fat, calories and sugar.
Baking Substitutions
Swap pureed prunes for butter, which have 50% less calories and fat than butter. Use this for dark baked goods, like brownies. Mix 3/4 cup prunes with 1/4 cup boiling water and puree to blend. Substitutes in equal amounts for butter.

Swap 1 cup of drained pureed black beans for 1 cup of flour in brownie recipes.

Add shredded zucchini to baked goods.

Add mashed fruit, like apricots and bananas that are naturally sweet instead of sugar to cakes, muffins, breads and cookies.

Swap oil for equal amounts of pureed fruits and vegetables in muffin, cookie and cake recipes.
It certainly will not happen overnight, but, with a little diligence and discipline it can be done and years later your child may even thank you for instilling habits that will serve them well into adulthood.

Encourage Exercise

There is a reason that obesity rates in kids have tripled since the 1960s and one of the biggest is that kids don't play outside like they used to. Technology with all its good has its negatives and one of those is that kids plug in from the time they get home and the physical activity they need daily suffers.
Even though the computer wins hands down as being the greatest invention of the 21st century it's also made children as well as many adults, lazy.
Children love computer games and can sit for hours and hours playing. They play with other friends or they even play with others across the country or across the world because the Internet lets us communicate with people from anywhere.
But, all that sitting is doing nothing for your child's health regimen. Toss in a pizza, bag of chips and soda, and that all night video game marathon just went from bad to worse, especially, if your child is overweight.
As parents and it may be difficult because the situation may have spiraled out of control, we must learn to put our proverbial foot down. If your child's weight has turned into a problem, it's up to the parents to initiate some rules and more importantly stick by those rules. It might be hard but it's easier when they're young to try to steer them onto the right path.

Studies have shown that many do not get nearly enough, and spend most of the day in sitting positions, while in school and after, playing video games and watching television at home.

Tips To Get Kids Active

Introduce activities that the family can do together, such as, baseball in the park, bowling in the winter or swimming in the summer.

Limit computer and video game time to either weekends only, or to set hours daily. Engage the whole family in fitness, by creating activities that get you outdoors. Schedule a 'game night' weekly and make sure to have fresh fruit salad and cut-up veggies with dip handy too.

Engage other families in the neighborhood to create "fitness play dates" where different parents can supervise on a set schedule, this can help with busy schedules when both parents work.

Set up a reward system or a gold star board for fitness achievements. Children respond really well to positive reinforcement. Setting up some type of reward system will encourage them to stay active.

Gold star boards that teachers often use in the classroom are great ideas for daily achievements. You can also go further and provide rewards, like special outings, or toy gifts for major achievements, such as, one month straight of daily physical activity. **Try not to use food as a reward, this makes kids associate food with other than its intended purpose, which is nutrition.**

Exercises For Kids

- Tag
- Structured sports (check your local YMCA and local little leagues)
- Set up competitive relay games where prizes are handed out to winners
- Fun obstacle courses, similar to those the military uses to train, can be set up in the back yard (make sure they are age appropriate)
- Running or walking challenges or meets between parents and siblings. A little healthy competition goes a long way to motivate kids and it is fun too!
- Walking family pets
- Mini trampolines
- Hiking
- Biking
- Running
- Swimming
- Cement chalk games
- Dancing
- Jumping rope
- Various outdoor games: Badminton, volleyball, basketball, slip and slides, and others, just check the toy and sporting goods aisle...

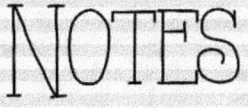

NOTES

Helping An Obese Child

Effects Of Obesity On Children

- Obesity in kids can lead to Type 2 diabetes, hypertension, early heart problems, high cholesterol, high blood pressure, and bone problems are and other related conditions.
- It can cause sleeping problems, body aches, acne, and loss of energy and stamina.
- A big side effect is that children have self-esteem issues often caused by negative body image and relentless teasing at school among their peers.
- They may be bullied in school or be acutely conscious of their body and feel different to other children and this might result in secondary problems like depression, stress, anger issues, inability to adjust to different situations, withdrawal and an inferiority complex.

Into Adulthood

In the long run, it has been noted that overweight children also go on to become overweight adults. The psychological problems persist and may transcend into more tangible forms like drug abuse, alcoholism, etc. Physical problems also arise in adults such as heart disease, cancer, osteoarthritis, diabetes, stroke, and shortened life expectancy. Inactivity, a habit garnered during the growing up years also manifests itself in adult life.

Children who preferred video gaming and television to sports may continue being couch potatoes in their adult life as well. This lifestyle is extremely harmful not only for the person but also friends and family close to him as it may lead to alienation and distance between people.

Dealing With Obese and Overweight Kids

Parents know their children best. They are the first ones to get any indication that something is not right. They are also aware of the family history and roots. Dieticians maintain that hormonal and genetic problems may also lead to children becoming overweight.

In such cases, parents need to be extra careful from the beginning to ensure that the child maintains a healthy lifestyle which includes proper full meals at mealtimes, healthy snacks, and loads of exercise in terms of extracurricular activities and sports.

For children, who are continuously growing, losing a bit of baby fat isn't as difficult as it is for adults. A few subtle changes will have major effects in a short while.

The thing to keep in mind is to not do anything too drastic. Instead slowly easing into the problem, and tackling it subtly, is the best course of action.

Lastly, it is important to be inclusive of everyone in the family and not single out one child for his/her weight issues or problems. This may do more harm than good.

So where do you start?

8 Steps To Making Changes

Love

Always come from a place of love and support. Offer encouragement and positive reinforcement for even the smallest of achievements in weight loss or exercise. **Read THE POWER by Rhonda Byrne if you need help in being more loving.**

Seek Help And Support As Needed

There are plenty of good nutritionists and dieticians to help you and your child. However, **it is best that you handle the meetings with them as there is a high chance that children might get demoralized with regular visits to doctors and dieticians.** Make sure to get a set weight loss plan with the correct amount of calories and the foods that are appropriate for your child. They are still growing and so require a certain amount of nutrition, so it is imperative that they lose weight the right way.

Know Your Child

Sometimes weight gain may have a physical or psychological aspect. Do some investigation, and consult with a physician as soon as possible. If your child is going through something, he/she may be diverting the energy and emotions into food. If that is the case, then address the problem at its root. Once the issue is resolved, your child will go back to his/her normal lifestyle and shed the weight he gained. If the problem still persists, consult a child psychologist.

Don't Blame

The worst thing to do is be accusatory and blame them for weight gain. Statements, like "I told you to stop eating all that ice cream" will not help anybody. And, these types of statements can do more harm than good because they can add to an already fragile and damaged self-esteem.

Deal With Teasing Issues

You can safely assume that if your child is obese or overweight they have been teased at school. Kids can be very cruel and thoughtless and teasing hurts, especially kids who do not have the coping mechanisms to deal with such pain and attention.

It's important that your child know that they can talk to you, and tell you what's going on. And, the effects of teasing must be dealt with. Often, kids are overweight and get teased begin to use food as a coping mechanism, which only propagates obesity. If you feel it necessary, it's okay to seek professional help in this regard too.

Be Tactful

Never be too direct as it may make your child run away from the problem and cause more eating problems. Ask pertinent questions about your child's lifestyle.

Children, especially teenagers like making their own decisions. So instead of dictating sermons, let them understand what the problem is. With careful guidance, you can help them arrive at conclusions and decide the next course of action.

Include The Whole Family

Singling out a child in the family is not the answer. You are a family and a family runs and works as a unit and so the entire family must get involved in the fitness and weight loss plan. Plus, a healthy lifestyle is beneficial to all.

So instead of saying you need to exercise more, start by taking up a hobby like dancing which requires a physical effort and then get your child involved. Get the whole family outside to run, play and be active.

This will provide you with more family time as well and allow you to bond with your child while helping him or her lose weight.

Meals should be the same for everyone.

If, traditionally there are unhealthy foods in the home they should all be removed. Meals should be prepared with health in mind and all snacks should be healthy, really, for everyone's sake, not just the child that needs to lose weight.

Be Age Appropriate

While younger children will listen to your commands, there is no need to bring them up to speed about their body all the time.

Let them have fun and under your supervision lose their weight. Teenagers like honesty so broach the issue upfront, but do not be accusatory or demanding. Instead be a friend to them and make decisions together. Join them in this effort and see the difference.

Set Short Term Goals

Children lose motivation and willpower easily. Since with children, rigid diets and hard core exercise is not the option, the results too are gradual. They need to be healthy first and weight loss will happen on its own accord. Therefore, be innovative in setting your goals.

For example, in children under the age of 10, make it fun by telling them that you will be measuring the speed at which they can run and the amount of time they take to complete 200 meters. Use a stop watch and make it a fun game. Join in as well. It will develop a healthy spirit of competition in the child along with being a challenge that they can easily conquer.

Consistent Meal Times

Ensure that your child eats his/her breakfast and finishes her lunch or snack that you have packed. Skip the junk foods and take some time out to cook. Make eating out a treat reserved for once a month. I have my twins read a book while waiting in a restaurant for our meals, and let them know that if they finish their entrée **and** accompanying fruit or yogurt, *then* they can have one scoop of ice cream.

This schedule applies for everybody. Once your child sees the level of dedication that everyone is putting in on his/her behalf, he/she will start putting in effort into shedding the extra weight.

Make Small Changes

Start with small changes and slowly move up the ladder. Children respond to this better.
You act as the messenger, seek their help and make the action happen.

With these steps, in a very short while your child will be back on track with a normal BMI and will be leading a happy and satisfied life.

I have created a Pinterest board with helpful information here:
www.pinterest.com/petralovesbats/childhood-obesity
Yes, I really do love bats.

Access your free report, The Most Fattening Foods and Healthier Substitutions for You and Your Child here:
http://gum.co/FatteningFoods

And I welcome your comments, feedback and honest review here:
www.amazon.com/author/petra

Now don't just stop reading this book and do nothing: take action now to get you and your child on the right track. I wish you well.

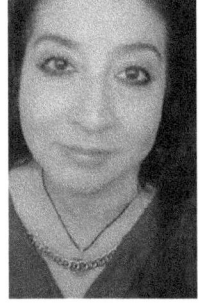

Petra

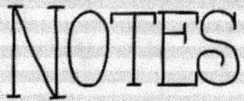

NOTES

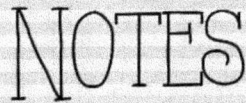

NOTES

NOTES

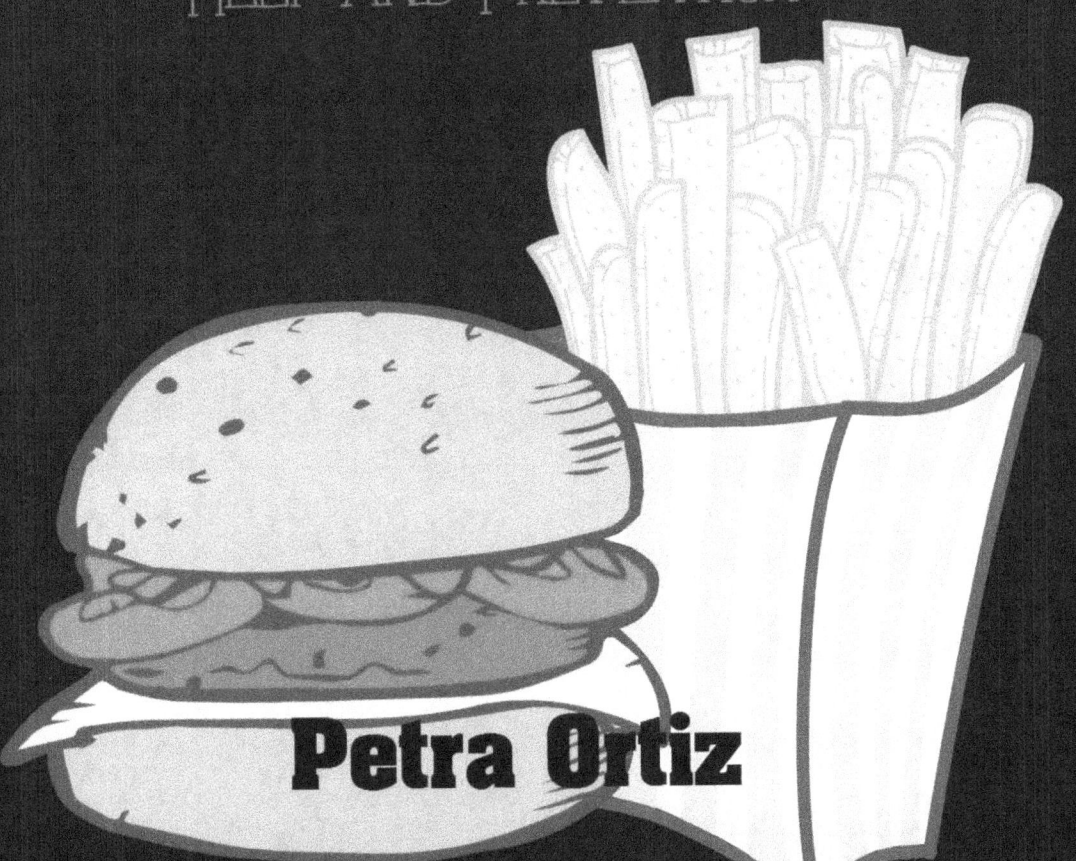

ADULT AND CHILDHOOD OBESITY

IMPACT, CONSEQUENCES, HELP AND PREVENTION

Petra Ortiz